Advance

Empty Hands ...

infertility with unashamed transparency and vulnerability. It is penned by one who shares with credibility and authority, drawing from her own personal journey.

Those who identify with the terms "childless," "infertile," or "child-free" will find solace in reading that another has traversed a similar road. Despite this, the author directs the reader to define who they are apart from these terms, to celebrate what is found, and to always return to the place of peace and rest. I recommend, encourage and challenge you to allow Paula to sincerely and lovingly show you how!

—Jennine Grant B.Sc.N., R.N., R.H.N.
Registered Nurse, Registered Holistic Nutritionist

Insightful and revealing... Paula has done a superb job sharing her journey through the valley of unfulfilled desire to find rest and peace in the green pastures of acceptance. Her intimate sharing from her heart will be an inspiration and encouragement to one who is hurting and seeking meaning when the deepest longing of the soul seems to be out of reach. Paula has discovered joy, peace, and wisdom which comes from learning to accept what she cannot change and do what she is able to with passion and joy... to love and care for the many precious children in her world and minister to them with a mother's heart.

— Pastor Robert Powell
New Beginnings Church, Alliston, ON

It has been my privilege to know the author for the past thirty years. The story she shares is true and a must-read for those who have found themselves in trying and challenging circumstances. Life does not always grant us every desire of our heart; sometimes we must make an adjustment and accept God's will. This book reveals the secret of how she came to accept what she could not change and the discoveries she made along the way. I recommend this book for today's generation.

—Pastor Gwyn Vaughn
Faith Christian Assembly, Seal Beach, CA

Empty Hands to Open Arms

From Infertility to Possibility

Run into His open arms!

Paula Hernando

Paula Hernando

Jesus, You never left my side. I'm forever grateful.
Dario, my best friend, you loved me enough to stay.
Every day I love you more.
My Novak parents and family.
You will always be fondly remembered, cherished, and celebrated.
To all the courageous women who believe
ten little fingers and ten little toes are worth it all.

Special Thanks

Pastors Bob and Brenda—your encouragement, love, and prayers paved my way.

Peter and Jan—you continually encouraged me to "use my words"!

To all the heart-grown children in my life, thanks for letting me love you for a time.

Table of Contents

IN MEMORY OF CASSIA   xi

Baby Wishes   1
Finding God   9
Infertile   17
Obsession for Love   21
Meeting, Courting, and Falling in Love   25
A Treasured Symbol of Love   27
A Room with a View   31
The Queen of Trying Hard   35
Heartfelt or Headfirst   41
The Empty Nest   47
Another Childless Mother's Day   49
Found Children   53
No More Wait in Me   57

PICTURES   64

From Mother to Mother   67
Lost and Found   73
The Other Mother   75
Assumptions   77
Beware of the Little Clouds   81
Living Child-Friendly   85
Who Am I to Become?   89
Such a Simple Question   91
This Is It!   93

Looking Back   97
Empty Hands to Open Arms   101
I See You Everywhere: An Imagined Scenario   103
If You've Ever Wondered   107

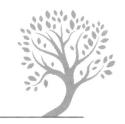

In Memory of Cassia

It was the eyes that caught your attention first. Those big brown eyes had so much understanding, mixed with love. In those eyes you could almost see her brief history of joy and hope, goodbyes and hellos, fears and comfort. She had shoulder-length red hair, a mixture of her grandmother's (on my husband's side) and my great-grandmother's, as well as highlights of my own blonde hair from when I was a child, like warm cinnamon. Her mouth relaxed in an almost tangible smile, guarded and shy, but emerging with each new day. Cassia's small rounded nose wrinkled at the way-too-healthy smell of broccoli. This was an opinion Cassia and I shared strongly.

Her voice carried a soft but high tone, in the way all children's voices do. At times her high-pitched cries would have you bolting to the rescue only to find that a small ant had struggled up her knee and was now peering dangerously at her. Other days, we'd smile at her funny way of singing her own songs of flowers and bumblebees. The little soft coos of "Mama" or "Daddy, wuv you" would melt our hearts. These moments touched us deeply.

Around her tiny right baby finger was wrapped all our intentions to spoil her, in that we could do her no harm and we would give her all she could possibly need in this world.

We gave her the name Cassia Elsa Emily. She was named after her grandmothers. The name Cassia is derived from a beautiful flower that in biblical times was used primarily as a spice in the oil for anointing kings and their garments. It smells like cinnamon; with red hair, the name fit Cassia perfectly.

Cassia is my child, my husband's and my little girl, conceived only in our imagination, affectionately loved in our dreams, teasingly named "Cassia Cookies" by my husband. She has been imagined often and spoken about continually in those first few early years of dreaming about conception. She was the imaginary creation of our hoping hearts. She has been lost forever. In our minds and hearts she is real, but we will never get to meet her.

Here is my story, as my husband and I journeyed together on this road of infertility. It offers hope when there seems to be no resolution, no answer. I write to those of you who are at the end of yourselves, having waited your lives away. Childlessness was never my plan, but it has been the road I travelled. My invitation to you is to grab a coffee, come, and sit a while, read a bit. The names have been changed to protect identities, but the emotions are real. For those of you who know this road, I trust you will find encouragement and peace—and that you will know you are never alone.

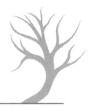

Baby Wishes

My parents, Emily and George, raised their family of seven children in rural Saskatchewan in the 1950s to the mid-70s. Our farm had much land where my father grew acres of wheat and raised cattle for our family's needs. Dad always worked hard and instilled fairness and hard work in the three boys of our family. I was the youngest of four daughters.

I have always been short in stature... actually, very short in stature. As an infant, I was diagnosed as a tiny, underweight "failure to thrive" baby. I was moved by ambulance to Regina to spend two to four months. My family had a new sibling, and my parents had a new baby, but I was hospitalized and I couldn't come home.

My mother raised us girls all the while managing the family garden, milking the cows, and cleaning and washing and cooking. As a young child, I followed her around, often asking her questions. I let everyone know that having a baby was all I ever wanted. It was my heart's greatest wish.

"Mommy?" I asked.

My mom paused in the middle of milking our dairy cow. "Yes?"

The cow she was milking turned her head just then to listen in.

"When do you think I could buy a baby?" I asked. "How much do they cost?"

Mom laughed at the thought. "You cannot buy a baby with money. A baby will come to you once you are married. It's better when you are older."

I didn't want to wait until I was older. I wanted one now.

My first baby doll arrived Christmas morning when I was five. That Christmas Eve, our tiny farmhouse was dark in the midnight hour. The moon held its place as the only illumination for a little girl determined to peek under the Christmas tree, just once.

I slipped out of bed as my Mom, Dad, and four older siblings slept in their respective rooms. My oldest brother and sister had already left home.

The shadows in the living room were a bit frightening. The potted philodendron in the corner loomed large with shadowy fingers that threatened to grab me as I passed. I was determined to follow the ribbed edge of the couch along the far wall, slip around the coffee table, and head straight toward the picture window. Our Christmas tree stood there with all its former glitter and lights now dim in the darkness. I crept forward, hardly breathing, afraid I would wake Mom or Dad. In the shadow, I reached out to touch a small baby carriage under the tree. The shape and feel of the pram was cold in my little hand. I felt inside for the tiny dolly that was sure to be there. The paper crumpled at my touch. As I peeked under the tree at this small wonder, I let out a squeal and my heart was lit!

When I opened my present later, I found my "baby." She wore a pink and white frilly dress, soft white socks, and tiny white plastic shoes. Her hair was short and blonde, and her eyes were a pretty blue with lids that opened and shut depending on how she was held. Pink lips pursed in smile, telling me she was glad to be home. Her arrival was complete with a blue and white carriage. I would hold my baby girl and smile. To me she was real, tangible, and in my own world, the fulfilled longing of a Christmas wish.

That longing to be married and have a baby would follow me throughout childhood. I simply loved children. I knew that one day I would be married. Like all children, I practised walking down the imaginary church aisle, holding my grandmother's geranium as a beautiful wedding bouquet. I smiled as I slipped on a green plastic twist-tie, fashioned into a ring. My plan always included my baby doll. That baby doll was so needy. An afternoon flew by with all the work of changing a diaper, feeding, bathing, and singing lullabies. In the late 60s, it was commonplace for girls everywhere to get married and have families. I understood in my young mind that to get a baby meant getting a boy, too. I didn't think it was too hard to do.

Most of my elementary years were filled with modified equipment to accommodate my needs. When I started school in Grade One, I was given an old wooden desk with a lift lid top; the legs were cut down so my feet could reach the floor. In the girl's bathroom, the last toilet had a semi-permanent potty seat that fit onto the toilet for my usage. A wooden step was built for me to reach the toilet seat, and another one helped me reach the hallway water fountain. As I got a bit older, I was assigned a small child's desk mounted on a wooden platform so my desk would be level with the other kids' desks.

As a preschooler, I could drive my tricycle under the kitchen table with quite a bit of clearance for my head. At six years of age, I was only twenty-five pounds. However, I carried on in my elementary years, oblivious to the growing concern of my family physician. My parents were made aware of his concern and told my parents of his intention to send me to Sick Kids Hospital in Toronto. In my father's words, the doctor said, "There's an experimental treatment that seems to be gaining a lot of approval using human growth hormone in children who cannot produce their own. There would be tests to see if Paula is eligible. I'd like to send her to a children's endocrinologist there."

"Can you guarantee that this treatment will work if we send her there?" my dad asked. The doctor shook his head. "Then I don't want my daughter to be a guinea pig."

My dad spoke with determination, and that was that.

It wasn't until many years later that I heard about this conversation. It came as a surprise when I learned of it in my doctor's office, during a routine appointment.

"Come in and sit down, Paula," Dr. Wallis told me.

I entered and climbed up onto the leather chair. My feet dangled as I pushed myself back into the seat. My throat burned with what was surely strep, and I felt like I needed to lie down. At twelve years of age, although I was small, I was becoming quite independent and had just spent the morning with my mom at her housekeeping position at a local hotel. We had just moved to this small town the year before, after selling our farm.

"What seems to be the problem?" He smiled and adjusted the stethoscope over his neck.

I complained about my painful throat. After a swab and a prescription for an antibiotic, I rose to leave.

Mom will have to give me money so I can pay for the prescription, I thought to myself. *If I hurry back to the hotel, then to the pharmacy, I can make it home in time to watch* Gilligan's Island—

"How old are you now?" Dr. Wallis asked.

The interruption startled me. "Twelve," I said.

He rose and walked over to the wall where the steel height rod was attached. "Let's check your height."

I obeyed and removed my shoes without being told. My height and weight measurement was common practice when it came to doctors' visits. At that point, I hadn't yet lived with the shame and teasing of being extremely short for my age. Junior High would prove to be more painful than I could imagine at twelve and a half. At only four feet tall, I hadn't yet been trapped in a school locker or hoisted to a back room cupboard and had the door forced shut. The teasing and nicknames—

like Tattoo and Millimetre—and songs ("Short people got no reason to live," they would sing) hadn't yet bruised my heart.

Dr. Wallis hesitated as he wrote some notes in the file. "I think it's time we send you to a specialist to see why you're not growing. I'll arrange for a referral and we will get to the bottom of all this."

Within six months, I was sitting in the office of Dr. R.M. Best, head of Endocrinology at the University Hospital in Saskatchewan. His assistant had the pleasure of taking my medical history. For a twelve-year-old, a three-hour history discussion with my parents was near torture. I didn't understand the magnitude of what was happening. I was registered as an outpatient, and for the next three days I was photographed in the nude, manipulated, tested, had blood work drawn, measured, weighed, poked, and prodded. Without explanations of all that was done, I felt violated. I wanted to go home!

Dr. Best was the greatest endocrinologist in the province. He was very matter-of-fact and told it exactly as it was. As he set out to explain his findings to my parents, I found myself confused. He used words like "pituitary disorder," "growth hormone supplementation," "anterior hypopituitarism," and "no tumour found."

Hypopituitarism is a rare disorder with the pituitary gland. In my case, the anterior of the pituitary had failed to produce the hormones necessary for growth. This tiny bean-shaped gland positioned at the underside of my brain, behind the nose, simply didn't work. I was described as a unique case, as I'd had no infections at birth, there were no tumours of the pituitary, and nothing was genetically wrong. The hypothalamus, which produces hormones of its own that directly affects the pituitary, worked perfectly. The cause, and therefore a cure, was unknown.

The specialists arranged for me to take a human growth hormone that would be injected three times a week for six months. Then I'd be given a six-month rest before resuming treatment. The hormone was extracted from the pituitaries of human cadavers. This practice continued through the 1960s to the late 80s, eventually being replaced with a synthetic recombinant growth hormone. Recombination was the process of molecular cloning to manufacture a protein that was nearly identical to naturally occurring human growth hormone. My parents were hopeful that this new treatment would enable me to live a happy and healthy life. I didn't want to be short into my adulthood, much less my teen years.

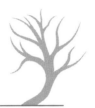

Finding God

The TV miniseries *Jesus of Nazareth* came out in 1977 at Easter, and although I had been raised in a church, I had never encountered a Jesus that seemed as real as this series portrayed. The actor Robert Powell gave an amazing re-enactment of the life, death, and resurrection of Jesus. I was mesmerized and sat glued to the television over the few days it aired.

As a child, I'd always had an awareness of God and would wander through the fields and wooded areas of our farm singing "He's got the whole world in His hands" and "Jesus loves me" at the top of my lungs. I always felt near to God and, although unaware of what it was called at the time, I sensed His presence. I believe these experiences were preparing me to meet Jesus, and the God who was calling me to Himself.

That summer, I looked forward to what every child waited for all year long: the summer exhibition, complete with food vendors, midway rides, games of chance, and local exhibitors. While my parents wandered off seeking displays of washing machines and farm equipment, I strolled through the colourful displays of a nearby building. I was told by my parents in no uncertain terms to stay inside this building. I obeyed and wandered around for over an hour. I found myself attracted to a table with colourful pictures of children. Over the back wall was a banner that read "Child Evangelism Fellowship." Being alone, I was a bit leery of moving in too close. I was attracted to the books and pamphlets there.

"Hello there! What is your name?" the lady behind the table said to me.

"Hi… um, Paula."

"Well, welcome. Here are some storybooks you might like."

She seemed kind enough and I felt suddenly at ease. She leaned forward as I took a step toward the table. I peered at the storybook and decided I really did like it. The problem was that, at thirteen years old, I only had enough money for the hot dog I was going to get later. I shook my head.

The lady, whom I learned years later was an associate of CEF, smiled again and reached to pick up a brochure. "Here's something you can take home. You can read it and then, when you are finished, you can pray the prayer at the back."

The title of the brochure was *Am I Too Little?* I quickly folded the tract, pushing it into my front pocket.

Later, as I waited in the car for my parents at the grocery store, I pulled out the wrinkled yet glossy paper. I read the story about a little girl who wanted to give her heart to Jesus, but felt she was too little. I couldn't wait to get to the last page to pray the prayer:

> Dear Lord Jesus, I know that I have sinned and I am truly sorry for my sins. I thank You for loving me so much and for dying on the cross for my sins, and rising again. Please come into my heart and be my Saviour.[1]

My head was bowed and my hands were folded as that same quiet peace filled my heart.

Time passed and that quiet presence drifted to the back of my teenage brain. I hadn't found anyone to walk me through my new faith, so I carried on in Junior High. I soon found three girls who wanted to hang out with me. We formed a small club of sorts, calling ourselves "the Cats," although we never actually owned any cats. We also loved Shaun Cassidy, a teen singer who had won our hearts.

For three years, I felt that these were the best friends I could have ever made. There was something so free, so wonderful about those years. In many ways, we were still children trying to figure out how to grow up, and at the same time enter the teenage drama that thrust us out of our childhood states.

We endured together through our first boyfriends and through our first experiences of the female "gift." The latter never came for me. I remember feeling like I'd been eliminated from a certain club that was awarded to girls everywhere, except for me.

---

[1] *Am I Too Little?* (Saskatoon, SK: Western Tract Mission, 2009), 6.

These were the years when I endured much teasing. The word "teasing" seems very non-threatening, yet what I endured as a young teen confirmed the self-repugnance I was beginning to feel in myself. I was a quiet girl and felt like I couldn't do anything right. I began to feel a deep inability to succeed. I struggled in mathematics, and buried my thoughts in books and became an avid reader.

During Junior High, our class was competing in a turkey trot. If you haven't heard of that, it's when a group of people come together for a fun run or a race, usually of the long-distance variety, held on or around Thanksgiving Day. My homeroom teacher thought this would be a fun way to get all the students out in the brisk air for some exercise. My height at the time was approximately 4'5" and I didn't have a lot of endurance and strength. I remember crying that I couldn't do it and was put on a modified run.

I began to feel that my height was a curse and became increasingly embarrassed that I couldn't do a lot of things the other kids could. Running in track and field, high jump, and long jump were especially embarrassing as these were marked by one's ability in distance and height. The steel bar was always dropped lower when my turn came. The teacher never bothered to measure my distance in long jump, and running just became a chance to take my turn rather than really compete. I learned to laugh it off with the other kids, but inside I was breaking.

Al Branchuk, my homeroom teacher and gym instructor, noticed my frustration and had a chat with me in the hallway. I was mortified. I thought I was in trouble.

"Your Mom called me last night, Paula," he said. "I guess you've been pretty upset about school. What's going on?"

I paused and looked up at this man whom I idolized in secret. I always wanted his attention but felt shy in trying to get it.

"Nothing really," I said. "I don't like it when the big kids call me names and some of the boys lock me in the locker."

That whole morning I was allowed to spend time in the library, where I browsed the stacks. My teacher was having a heart-to-heart with the kids in our classroom at the time. I never found out what he said, but my heart marvelled that he would take the time to care.

I was always looking to belong. My parents found new jobs when we moved to Moose Jaw in the spring of 1980. All I thought I needed was a friend. Having had to leave all my good friends in our community, I longed for someone to hang out with. From my experiences in Junior High, it was a big hole to fill.

The pattern of my injections—six months on, six months off—became habitual and I didn't give it much thought. Certainly I didn't like it. The three-time weekly injections always stung a little, but they didn't seem to trouble me in the three years I had followed the program thus far.

September came and I found my Grade Ten English class after registering in the school counsellor's office. I took a middle row seat, drew a deep breath, and sat down.

The girl in front of me turned around to gaze at me. "Hey, guess what?"

"What?" I said, trying to smile and look friendly.

"I got saved last night!" As this girl spoke, her eyes beamed with joy.

"From what?"

She couldn't answer just then, as our teacher had walked into the room. As he began the morning lesson, I pondered what this girl had meant.

Later, I discovered that Victoria had, just the night before, accepted Jesus into her heart. Although I had forgotten the prayer in my parent's car years before, something gnawed at me. Something inside me wanted to belong, too, to listen as Victoria excitedly shared her faith with me.

The conviction of being disconnected from God led me to find my parents' family Bible. For two weeks, I read and reread the book of Revelation. It demonstrated to me the awesome power of God, and at sixteen it really freaked me out. Every night I knelt by my bed and prayed, "Dear God, if I am not saved, would you please save me and come into my heart? Thanks."

I never had complete assurance until the night I attended Crossroads Coffeehouse in Moose Jaw. This happy hangout was for teens to enjoy music, fellowship, and coffee and donuts. I loved it there immediately. I had told my friend Victoria that I, too, was saved. Although I didn't have the assurance at the time, it was indeed true.

One night a group of teens decided to go into the park to sing and pray. I followed Victoria and tried to sing along.

My heart was filled with guilt. *You're lying and these people don't know it,* I thought. *Are you saved? Really, are you saved?*

"Victoria, I have to tell you, I'm not really saved. I mean, I don't think I am born again. I don't know Jesus. I'm sorry I didn't tell you the truth." By then, tears had started to stream down my cheeks.

Victoria put her hand on my shoulder. "Well, do you want to?"

I nodded and she asked another boy, John, to join us in prayer. He was a taller teen and very zealous when it came to the things of God. John smiled as he pulled out a gospel tract called *The Four Spiritual Laws.* As John led me through the tiny booklet, all I could think was how we could get through it faster.

When we finally prayed, I felt the dread and condemnation lift off my heart. I felt lighter and somehow in tune with God. Things were going to be different now!

I sensed hope as my hand turned the doorknob of my parents' home.

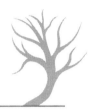

Infertile

Hope didn't last very long. Things didn't seem to work out the way I'd thought they would. I seemed to plummet into weepy instability and depression.

This emotional mess continued throughout my life in varying degrees and well into adulthood. Many troubles seemed to follow me with my family relationships, school shyness, painful teasing, and a deep sadness I couldn't shake. I had begun a pattern of self-loathing and even donned a t-shirt that said "God don't make junk" in an effort to feel better about myself.

I longed for more independence as a high school graduate. At eighteen, I'd had my share of hiccups, but I was learning to trust God for the simple things, like a job and finally my own apartment.

I opted to conclude my growth hormone injections after high school. Dr. Best wasn't pleased at this independent decision, but my parents had given me the choice now that I was eighteen. I could make my own decisions about my life.

Much to my parents' dismay, I began to attend Victoria's church and made many friends there. I learned about what the Bible had to say about my life and even read the stories of Ruth and Mary. Their stories inspired my desire for marriage. Friends all around me had relationships, got married, and had babies. Where was my dream come true? I also read about Elizabeth, Hannah, and Sarah, and their longing for restoration from their barrenness. I never knew I was like them.

I can remember when I first heard the word "infertile" as an unsuspecting nineteen-year-old. I was unmarried and visiting my new doctor for investigation into why I hadn't reached puberty. While waiting for her to write a referral, she eyed me and blurted, "Oh, I guess you know with this condition of the pituitary, you cannot have kids. I suppose you know that you are infertile."

"No, I didn't know that," I responded.

I was sort of dumfounded. If there was a course for my doctor to have taken called "How to Tell a Patient She Is Infertile," she had obviously missed that class. No one, not one doctor in all my years of seeing them, had mentioned this. I felt betrayed.

It was the cruellest joke. For my whole life, I'd been on course to one day, after marriage, literally hold my dream in my arms. I wanted a child, but now I had a diagnosis of infertility. I cried that night, even though my doctor had called my parents to ensure I would be all right.

Where was the compassion? Where was the solution, or resolution? I couldn't go for any specific treatment to fix myself, because I wasn't married. I felt no one could understand.

Finally, after three days of hurting and wondering and feeling so lost, I told my brother Merv. We had worked together in the same grocery store and I felt safe with him. When I told him, he put his strong arm around me.

"Sorry, Kiddo."

I found this news devastating. An existing condition at birth would keep me from holding my own child. If hope deferred makes the heart sick (Proverbs 13:12), then hope dashed makes the heart break.

My prayers changed after that. Yes, I was still seeking to be married, but now I was asking to be healed. I wanted so much to be fixed. I felt so alone.

In time, it was determined that my condition included the need for replacement hormones. My body basically didn't make the basic hormones needed for reproduction, so I was put on a cyclical treatment of estrogen and progesterone. This explained some of my emotional ups and downs. Hormones such as follicle-stimulating hormone (FSH) and luteinizing hormone (LH) could be replaced by injection to stimulate ovulation once I married.

I knew I wasn't capable of conceiving, and now I had to deal with more hormone replacement therapy just to have a normal life. Not a pill-taker by nature, I bucked at the thought of having to deal with this forever.

The problem was that marriage didn't come until six months after my thirty-ninth birthday. It felt like the ultimate rejection. For anyone wanting a husband, it's a long time to wait twenty years. For me I knew—just knew—that if I could just be married, I would have all my yearnings met. Surely I would conceive, just because. I felt like I had paid my dues for waiting… but I had no idea what waiting really was. I was in denial of reality. I thought it would all work out somehow. I basically had assumed that I would receive a healing. I went to every healing line for prayer that I could, and I waited.

However, marriage was a long way away. For the next several years, I focused on the business of a new career in early childhood education. For two years I enjoyed learning about children, their development, and ways to inspire their learning. When I received my diploma, I plunged into work at childcare centres, became an educational assistant for the hearing-impaired, and enjoyed using my gifts as a children's church teacher. I had many children in my life, and while I enjoyed this type of work in the early years, my heart's cry was to have one of my own. I wanted to be married, and I wanted to have a child.

I saw that the only way I could achieve a pregnancy was if I had a husband. This became an obsession in every way, and it was a continual prayer to the Lord.

Obsession for Love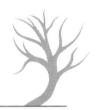

The next twenty years passed in a bit of a blur. Have you ever wanted to prepare in advance for something so much that you took an anything-goes approach? I did. I was preparing myself to be completely healed. There was no point in pursuing infertility treatment, as I was single. I wasn't prepared for the cost it would involve and for being a single mom if it worked.

One day at church, I felt that I got my answer. A special visiting speaker had the gift of uttering words from the Lord. I was called out and he prophesied over my future.

"I see lots of children," he said. "In children's ministry you'll do greater things than what you've already done. You will have a baby, babies from your own body. This could be the year that you'll find your man, or rather he'll find you, because if we [the church] wait for you, we'll wait forever…"

I couldn't contain my excitement! Now I knew that when I married, God would heal my body. I was so sure of it, so happy that there was hope. Time, however, proved slow in finding a man—or rather, him finding me. It was not one year, or two, or even three: still no man, and no babies. I sank once again into disappointment.

I wrote in my journal one morning while crying, weeping in my loneliness for affection, as I often did in my perceived need to be valued. I became demanding, wanting the Lord to do something to bring me my heart's desire. I was sure He could bring me a husband. I wrote,

> All people have a need within themselves to be significant, in relationship, in purpose or value. I want to be wanted. I want to give myself to someone in wanting them. To be valuable to someone, to be important to one other person, to be someone else's priority. There are times when I don't feel good enough or important enough to warrant anyone's attention, much less a man. Many times individuals always defer to someone else's agenda, interrupted because of someone else's louder need or importance, someone more prominent than they. Here I am all the while aching on the inside for my turn. When will I be someone's number one? When will I get to be put on your agenda with inerasable ink?

If you asked any of my friends "What does Paula want most?" they would probably answer, "To be married and have children." Of course I would love to be married, and of course I would love to have children, whether they be our own, his children, or children we adopted together. To me it seemed like a package deal. I longed to have the opportunity to exchange my single life challenges for married life challenges. My father used to tell me, "It doesn't matter if you're his first love, just make sure that you're his last."

Meeting, Courting, and Falling in Love

I got both… I was Dario's first and his last love. I met him in the fall of 1998, a season in which I took a break from working with children and decided to use my secretarial skills to assist at a Bible college in Saskatchewan. I aided from time to time with new student arrivals and worked with the people in the church to house students in room-and-board situations.

That morning, I heard from my employer that an individual would be arriving and needed housing while he was in the city and attending church. Once I contacted my list of landlords, I found an opening for this man.

I had prepared a "Welcome to Saskatoon" package, along with information on our church and college. It was a function I had repeated many times. Dario Hernando was set to arrive that afternoon, and I was ready.

I wasn't ready for the moment he walked into the front office. I remember so clearly stepping into the office foyer to see this tall, dark, and handsome man. The initial fluttering of my heart left me a bit flustered as I tried to hide my attraction.

I managed to get through. I may have blushed. After a moment or five, Dario was on his way to find his billet.

Over the next few years, Dario and I became good friends, acquaintances who never seemed too far apart during fellowship time after church or group events with friends. We always gravitated toward one another.

It was February 2003 when finally Dario asked me out to dinner. I was very nervous as we drove up to the Asian restaurant he'd picked out for us. I knew this was something special when I tried squid for the first and last time in my life.

Our courtship continued through spring and I knew Dario was "the one." We spent a lot of time together on coffee or dinner dates and often talked into the wee hours of the morning. Whenever possible, our conversations continued on the phone.

My roommates knew we were getting serious. I couldn't wait to marry Dario! I secretly hoped it would be soon, as I was ready to check "marriage" off my bucket list and then "baby" soon after. I dismissed the infertility diagnosis and assumed there'd be a miracle. For the time being, I was happy and content to visit places and enjoy day-tripping with my new love.

A Treasured Symbol of Love

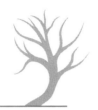

One of our many excursions brought us to Honeywood Heritage Nursery in Saskatchewan. I had anticipated visiting this dazzling piece of restored property. The day lilies, peonies, lilacs, plum, and rhubarb, and even apples and crab apples, were part of the horticulture of prairie days past. Today was the day my boyfriend and I planned to visit these gardens.

I remember as a child picking up a special flower and pulling the petals off one by one, saying, "He loves me, he loves me not, he loves me..." This ritual was to give me the knowledge of a special someone's love. I think, for this reason, I have always loved flowers.

The warm sunshine on this Canada Day was beautiful as Dario and I set out for a wonderful day together and a hopeful picnic. I felt the excitement way down to my toes. I had been dating this wonderful man for six months, but my heart for him had already been lit in friendship.

After the drive, we parked in the lot next to the swinging gate and met our tour guide. For the moment, our picnic lay cold and preserved in the car cooler. Dazzling whites, purples, reds, oranges, and bright sunshine yellow filled the green landscape of trees and shrubs. We learned of its history and how the many plants and flowers were hidden in the overgrowth of many years of neglect after the change of ownership. In later years, the beautiful nursery was lovingly restored. Tourism Saskatchewan and the Architectural Heritage Society of Saskatchewan recognized Honeywood's efforts for this cause.

The day turned hot and our gracious guide allowed us to use the small cabin for visitors to escape for a few moments to sign the guestbook and use the facilities. We set up to prepare for our table picnic. The birds chirped nearby in eager anticipation of what was about to happen.

I should have guessed that something was up when Dario began to put a camera and tripod in place. He had prepared red and white flowers in glass bowls, sparkling water to drink, wine glasses with red and white ribbon, and some tasty treats to add to our own summer sandwiches and coffee. It seemed a little over the top just for Canada Day.

My life was about to change through one special treasured object.

We seated ourselves at the table. Being hungry after our hike, I was eager to dig in. The cuisine looked so enticing and the sparkling water so refreshing, I could hardly believe when Dario told me to wait.

Seated next to me, Dario took my hand. "You know, Paula, I have really enjoyed the time we have spent together these past months. I have always treasured your friendship, too. I have found that I have fallen in love with you."

"Oh Dario," I replied, "I know, and I feel the same way, too."

Now can we eat, I thought.

With a half-smile, Dario bent down and got on one knee while fishing in his pocket for something and never losing his gaze with mine.

"You don't get it," he said.

With that comment he presented an open ring box with the most magnificent diamond ring inside it. The engagement ring was a solid gold band extending to a diamond-shaped gold base. Placed on the north and south rounded tips were two tiny diamonds. In the positions of east and west were medium-sized diamonds in a perfect trio, forming a heart. These diamonds nestled together with a large diamond in the middle, settled in a snug gold claw. The diamonds cascaded in what appeared to be a perfect waterfall.

These cut stones glistened and shimmered in the sunlight. The sparkle reflected what was sure to be seen in my watery eyes.

"I'm asking if you'll marry me."

Dario smiled and waited.

Joy burst through me and tears welled up as I nodded. A gentle kiss and warm embrace preceded the putting on of the ring. The diamond and gold were so much more beautiful than the simple twist-tie ring I had fashioned as a child, but the thrill was the same. It was exactly the same.

This ring would bring us through the great, the not-so-great, and the downright ugly times that only a committed marriage can know. This ring, my most prized object, came to represent all that love in the challenges that lay before us as husband and wife.

We were married on October 10, 2003, and we've never looked back.

In moments when life handed us disagreements, misunderstandings, and even infertility, the icon of our love has never lost its shine.

This is why my engagement/wedding ring has such value to me—and not just because it was a huge financial investment; a simple band would have meant the same to me. Dario once told me that this ring represented his love, but his actual love was so much greater. Though this ring represented that love, it was and is only an object. I can look at its beauty and remember, "He loves me, he really loves me." The real treasure on this earth for me is him.

A Room with a View

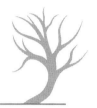

There are moments in time when, in the deepest place of your memory, you find the joy of a dream fulfilled.

It is October 2003, and I am softly awakened, remembering the joy of the previous four days. All the planning and organization that went into the wedding was worth all the tension. Our nine-month romance filled our days with phone calls, emails, and weeknight dates, culminating in long night talks.

Dario and I are newlyweds. I remember the ring, gold and diamond encircling my finger, and I smile. It's still so pretty. I'm still smiling as images and sensations of our first night together fill my mind and heart with the feeling of being so loved and cherished.

My eyes open slowly to view this room, in a condominium rented as a wedding present from the in-laws I have barely met.

Looking out the window, I drink in the beauty of the Hawaiian foliage as gentle winds and soft early morning rains refresh the tropical palms. The rain mists through my open window, dropping its precious spray directly to the ground. Amazingly, the screen remains dry. The window is framed with crème linen that billows in the breeze; each movement introduced a delicious refreshing zephyr.

The walls themselves are a pallet for the beautiful colours of this beloved island. Photos of Maui's tropical fruit trees, anthuriums, and orchids grace the four walls. Only yesterday I admired a painted protea flower. At this moment it's hidden from view. These art pieces invite me to explore the outdoors in the sunshine soon to come. But not just yet.

I turn in bed as I sense I'm alone. The first thing I see is the indentation in the pillow where only hours ago my husband lay his head. The sheets are rumpled around where he slept, but I'm not alarmed. The headboard is made from beautiful Koa wood forming a high triangular peak. The nightstands are a perfect match with two drawers each and brass handles. My eyes drift to the dressing table. Its elegance is unmatched, with curly patterns carved into the wood.

I remember that my new husband is on his morning walk to the beach just outside our door. Local merchants are gathering fresh produce and fruit for a daily sale, even in the rain. My husband has left me to rest, mindful of his promise of breakfast with toast, eggs benedict, and fresh mango.

I'm filled with contentment and anticipation for spending time with my love.

Unknown to both of us is that in a few short hours, tears will spill from my eyes as we discuss the hopes of a family and the realities of infertility. We will imagine together our firstborn, Cassia. This is where she was conceived in our imagination.

Lessons of value rarely come in the short trials of life. The lessons God allows us to meander through by our own choices often take years for the truth to set in, be understood, and bring change. They often come at a high emotional cost, causing us to spend every ounce of strength we have. God waits for such moments, for in these split seconds, He is there. It's exactly where He wants us to be, when we surrender and He enters in.

I always expected to be a mom. Many times, as a single person, I would bring the matter before God, praying to be healed. In my mind, if I could get things fixed up before I was married, voila! I could conceive on the wedding night! I had it all planned out. I was so convinced; I waited for all the signs. Month after painful month I waited, and I found that in fact those signs would never come. Our first years of marriage were bruised by the painful realities of infertility.

There was a broken place inside me. I wanted things to be just the way I had planned. I continually needed to know every detail, the why and how and when. I needed to be in control.

The Queen of Trying Hard

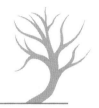

Our creative God, able to produce the most beautiful objects in nature, stands in stark contrast to me. I am unable to create even one small being. One small achievement for women has become something impossible for me. At times this thought saddened me in my deepest parts.

I was the queen of trying hard. During the first years after my diagnosis, and for the duration of our marriage, I hoped that somehow if I tried hard enough I would find the key to unlocking the healing I craved and was so desperate to achieve. I looked for solutions behind book covers, changed my diet, charted temperatures, took supplements, and even tried medication to bring about the wonderful marvel of pregnancy.

Dear God, please fix what is broken in me. This was a continual plea. I had wanted to be perfectly well before I was married. I was convinced I would conceive on our wedding night in 2003. When that didn't happen, I assumed that I would need medical help.

I added prayer to my "trying hard" regime, armed with Bible verses and books on receiving my miracle. I prayed, asked, and commanded, trying with all my desperation to bend the hand of God. In my error, I thought that if I proceeded with all the things that worked for others, and did them perfectly well, God would have to answer my prayers. If I did it all, *then* God would owe me a baby. I had heard that if I confessed enough, I would receive from God.

I prayed, "In Jesus' name, I receive strength to conceive seed. Pituitary, I command you to function perfectly the way you were created to function. I command you to release estrogen and progesterone in the proper amounts and at the proper time. I command you to release the follicle-stimulating hormone in the proper amounts and at the proper time to stimulate the ovaries to release a perfect, healthy, mature egg. I command you, body, to release the luteinizing hormone. I also command you to release growth hormone enough for my body and my baby's body at the proper intervals. Body, conceive and be pregnant! Your Word, God, says that none shall cast their young nor be barren among Your people. I thank You for the gift that will grow inside of me. You are so faithful in all that You promised us!"

I prayed and confessed and wept, daily, weekly, monthly… until I grew weary. The problem was, I didn't believe a word of it.

Each month, the single blue line on the pregnancy test screamed that it didn't work!

It was simple: I wanted a child, period. In fact, after I was married I poured over the details of my condition, learning everything about how a woman conceives a child, apart from the obvious. I delved into the processes of hormones, cell development, and how interruptions to the delicate process can make it all fail. My one thought was that if I could just figure out what the missing piece was, I could replace it with a reasonable facsimile and once again, voila, problem solved.

My husband and I attempted to get help and were referred to a reproductive gynaecologist, Dr. Chanen.

The day arrived when, with a hopeful heart, I sat in the office of my reproductive gynaecologist after undergoing many tests. My husband and I were hopeful that through modern medicine we could become pregnant through in vitro fertilization, or IVF. In this process, several eggs are harvested and united with male sperm outside of the body. This forced introduction is kind of like speed-dating at a dinner party. This appointment was to determine my eligibility.

I should have guessed something was wrong when my physician brought in a student psychologist to observe and assist in the appointment. The doctor's gentle deliverance of the news matched the gentle comfort of her assistant: "We're sorry, no." Due to complications of attempting pregnancy in my forties, the health risks, and the small percentage of success outweighing the incredible cost of each attempt, it was decided that I didn't qualify.

I couldn't speak. A tsunami of hot tears claimed me. I remember hearing that accusing voice: "You've failed, you've failed, you've failed." I was crushed, so crushed that I secretly vowed that having a child would have to be a miracle.

When Dr. Chanen announced that we didn't qualify for IVF treatment, she had sealed our fate in the medical sense. Without divine intervention, we would be childless. Although I wanted so desperately to give my husband a family he wanted, I couldn't do it. Although I yearned for a medical breakthrough to heal my body, it was not to come.

After several moments, I was ushered into a side room to gather myself before exiting the building. I would never go back.

I returned to the computer to pursue answers, found books that dealt with healing (in particular healing for infertility), and went to every healing prayer line I could find. I thought that if I did everything right and followed every direction set forth, God would owe me a child. I believed that because He had set up the system, He would be responsible for seeing it through. Anger and bitterness toward God grew inside me as I tried very hard to make happen what was not possible. I prayed, commanded, demanded, quoted Scripture to God, and basically told my body it would have to obey. I cried tears many times in complete helplessness and frustration. Why wasn't it working?

Oh how my heart ached for the fulfillment of a perceived promise. Didn't God owe me? Wasn't it normal to want what others so easily achieved? These empty hands were meant to be filled, weren't they? My arms ached to hold a little one, safely resting and trusting me to care for her every need, confident that she would not be dropped, hurt, or frightened. Is there any other place where this trust is so perfectly expressed than in the face of a sleeping child in her mother's arms? My heart ached for the gift given to every mother.

I finally let go of the idea that I would have a child through my own body. I still believed God owed me, though, so my husband and I decided to pursue adoption. The process seemed hopeful at the beginning, but delay after delay after delay brought about a deep hopelessness, and it damaged me.

No time ever seemed to be an appropriate time to begin the adoption process, but finally, in 2007, we began what would become a seven-year journey through paperwork, medical forms, and police checks.

I was excited when we had our first meeting with Children's Aid. We did what most couples do. We cleaned our house from top to bottom to make the best impression possible. I was beyond thrilled when it seemed that our dream of having a child could happen. Sure, it wouldn't be our own biological child, but it was certainly a child. Could we love someone else's child? We surely believed we could.

That meeting, with all its hopes and dreams, didn't result in the forward movement we had desired. In our interview, it was determined that our lives were too shaky for us to be considered candidates for adoption. We had gone through a lot in our first three years of marriage, and I had become emotionally fragile. Many things were revealed to us in that meeting about how we would have to heal and stabilize in order to move forward. I sobbed in sorrow, anger, and disbelief. Our file was put on hold and we waited. The news crushed us.

I continued to grieve through the years that followed. We set ourselves to a reinvention process whereby I received counselling, we further prepared our home, and we waited. We established a summer day camp for children and set up a playroom and fully prepped bedroom.

Finally, in 2011, we received a letter inviting us to attend the upcoming PRIDE (Parent Resources for Information, Development, and Education) classes. My husband and I were thrilled. Now could we have what our hearts had yearned for? Now were we ready? Now would we qualify? This thirteen-week class was a joy to be a part of and we felt that things were progressing rapidly. For us, the rain had stopped and the sun was shining again.

Following this process, we had an opportunity to begin our home study, and we were very nervous. Once again we cleaned our house from top to bottom. We completed, once again, all the required paperwork to update our file. We met with the original case worker who had met with us and began a series of meetings. During this process of meetings, we had everything ready in our home. One of the final goals in our reinvention process had been to eliminate some debt that we carried: we had to sell our home. We achieved our goal.

Even the sadness of moving out of our beloved home couldn't squelch that final announcement from Children's Aid. We'd made it. We were adoption-ready!

Heartfelt or Headfirst?

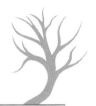

Sometimes the little things about infertility can come between a husband and wife. The following fictional scenario is an amalgamation of many conversations Dario and I had over the years we were seeking adoption. Those conversations almost always ended in frustration and tears.

* * *

Sarah passed through the hallway to the back bedroom where she knew her book and slippers awaited her. This had been a particularly difficult day with two children getting very sick in her preschool class. It wasn't the throwing up that made her so exhausted; it was keeping the entire classroom under control and getting help with the clean-up. She loved children, but this was not one of her better days.

She passed by the open door to a child's room and glanced inside. The bed, dresser, desk, and toy shelf, all made of maple, were arranged perfectly for a little one to play in. The curtains and bedspreads matched and the pillows had the same colouring as a beautiful bear tapestry hanging over the headboard. Sarah had come in here often in the early days, just to gaze at its arrangement and readiness for what was sure to be a home for her and her husband's little child. Adopting seemed like the perfect way to start a family.

"Hi, honey. Daydreaming again?"

Sarah turned to see her husband leaning in the doorway. Chris was tall and handsome and Sarah had fallen in love easily when she spotted him some eight years prior. A smile curved up Sarah's lips.

"What's so amusing, Sarah?" he asked. "Why are you in here again?"

"I'm just looking. I always wanted this room to be used, not sit empty like this. And I was smiling because you're home and I was just thinking how perfect some shelving would look right above the toy shelf. It would be great for the toys I bought the other day. What do you think?"

Chris paused before answering. "Oh Sarah, you know how much I want there to be a kid here, too, but we can't keep preparing a room for someone who we have no guarantee is coming. It's been five years since we applied to Children's Aid. Be realistic."

"Be realistic? I am being realistic." Sarah's heart pounded. She could feel her face getting hot. "You keep telling me that we don't have the money to continue this adoption, and I'm so frustrated. I would give anything to have this child, but I feel alone here. I've done all the paperwork and worked hard to get this room ready. If it weren't for me, we would never have come this far."

"This room could be utilized for other things. It could be our library. We still haven't unpacked books because we don't have space. Now listen, I was thinking, can we have this half of the room be a guest area? We could put up all the book shelves from the basement in the other half. We could take out the rocking chair and move in the small love seat. It would be comfortable and usable."

"No! We have to have this ready for our child. Don't you want one?" Sarah folded her arms and pushed away any conflicting thoughts of giving up her dream. She secretly couldn't bear to see what closing the door to Chris being a daddy would do to him. She knew what he really wanted.

"Of course I want one," he said. "We can put things in order when the time comes. I know that we need a great miracle in our finances if we can even be ready to receive a child. You keep buying things we don't need and spending money. Some things just have to happen first."

"You don't even care. You say you want to be a dad, but you're not willing to sacrifice for it. I can't believe you would just throw it all away." Sarah felt the hopelessness settle in the pit of her stomach and rise to her throat. She started to sob. "Don't you realize that this could be our last chance? We aren't getting any younger. If we're not ready now, when will we be ready?"

Chris winced. His pain wasn't aimed at the issue at hand; he'd managed to upset his wife once again. It always managed to be his fault. It always ended with Sarah in tears and Chris wondering what had happened. It was always about this room and the long wait for adoption. He wasn't sure how much more he and she could take.

"Sarah… calm down. Come here." Many arguments ago, Chris had figured out that the best way to handle these moments was to stop the disagreement and just hold her. The tears troubled him, but there wasn't much else he could do. Inside he was broken, too.

* * *

Marriages and relationships go through a terrible strain when there are infertility issues. Many of the drugs used to create an environment for pregnancy can have side effects and emotional highs and lows. Being able to communicate is so important for both spouses. The wife must be able to communicate what's going on and what she needs. The husband needs to know when to step back in order deescalate a situation and protect himself emotionally. At times, a comment such as "I know you're hurting right now and I'm here" is enough to quell a raging storm. Holding one another validates and communicates unspoken comfort.

I personally felt that I had failed Dario because I couldn't give him the child he wanted. We had many discussions around this theme, even after our engagement.

"I know you may not want to marry me," I had told him. "You know I cannot have kids. I know how much this means to you. I would be hurt, but I understand."

Dario always responded that we would work things out and do whatever we could. He often assured me of his love. Many times after we married and set up our little nest, we returned to this conversation.

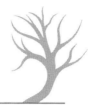

The Empty Nest

The paint on the bedroom wall is faded to a tired blue. A tiny shelf with a wooden helicopter and worn copy of *Goodnight Moon* sits alone, a faded copy of a well-loved tale fingered eagerly by other children. The matching desk and chest of drawers sit empty. The tapestry of a smiling bear hangs above a bed once full of the imaginings of little fingers and toes curled beneath the blue blanket once owned by a wannabe father, my husband.

I do not come in this room very much anymore. The sound of the ticking clock on the nightstand mocks the unheard cry in my own heart. It's too much to bear some days, the sounds of time spent waiting.

Another day is ending. I rush to the place of slumber until morning, where unhurried thoughts find their way into the quiet of my time alone in the early morning hours here, near my empty nest.

Waiting for all the proverbial ducks to get in a row has at times been the most painful thing. There are no crises in waiting, no reason to put you on an emergency prayer tree or for friends to ask how things are going. As the years progress and still no baby, it seems that even my husband has moved on and closed the parenting box in his mind.

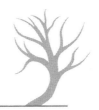

Another Childless Mother's Day

Mother's Day every year carried a tired dread, as I thought about it weeks in advance. What exactly do I think about in times like these? I know this: at my age, I've missed the opportunity to have my own child in the physical sense. Part of me knows that I no longer need to be pregnant, but another part of me is like that little kid who wants to cry out, "Pick me! Pick me!" I do long to give my love to a child. I want to be a mother, too! It's not that I'm jealous or angry; I've long worked past that.

In time, and with tears, came a type of forced surrender. It's just that I wanted to share the joys and frustrations of parenting, and I've been sad to have to wait so long for our adopted child to come.

In times past, I've wanted to hide—and at times I did. I just stayed in bed, pretending it was just another day. I would go about sorting laundry or restocking my bookshelf, meaningless things. I wanted to stay home… but even in that quiet isolation, I would realize that I wasn't having much fun. Finally in surrender, I planned to be others-focused and attempt to make Mother's Day about the mothers in my life, many who were cherished friends.

There were many Mother's Days when I felt I couldn't bear the hot flush of my cheeks, the inner embarrassment and voices that called out in my head, "Loser, failure, you don't belong." In times like these, God in His great mercy and compassion would move someone, often my pastor, Robert Powell, to offer prayer, hope, and consolation. He'd say, "God knows your deep desire and knows how to bring to pass His plans for you. I know your heart aches for a child, and I must say that our hearts ache as well, for we want so much to see God's hand move in your situation. The important thing is to achieve a peace which passes all understanding and to rest in God, knowing that even if our true heart's desire seems slow in coming, God loves us and we love Him. His ways are higher than our ways and His thoughts than ours. My wife and I continue to pray for you. God answers prayer in ways that surprise us and we are believing with you. We love you and Dario both, and you are dear to our hearts. Keep your eyes on Jesus and focus on the blessings that are all around you right now. You have not dropped the ball or failed in any way. You are not a mother from the traditional standpoint, but you have a mother's heart."

These were moments when my heart-cry to God seemed to go unheard. I would then turn often to my journal for a release of pain:

Dear Heavenly Father, this has been a rough week so far. The inability to have children has provoked in me determination, desire, hunger, tears, pain, and heartfelt prayers more than anything else in my life. I am so depressed about this hope deferred, and yes, Lord, I am heartsick. It's actually a physical pain in my very heart and soul. I have looked for you, Lord, to fulfill this desire in the last six and a half years of my marriage, but I've been asking you for a miracle for over twenty-five years… that was when I still had some hope and trust. I feel depleted of that hope, and at times I want to throw in the towel and give up completely on this life. Take me as I am, Lord, and restore me. Give me Your will and a sense of peace.

In these instances, the Lord did teach me. He showed me that He heard every cry of my heart, and I was learning to trust Him. He would speak to me quietly through verses like:

For I am the Lord your God who takes hold of your right hand and says to you, Do not fear; I will help you. (Isaiah 41:13, NIV)

The Lord himself goes before you and will be with you; he will never leave you nor forsake you. Do not be afraid; do not be discouraged. (Deuteronomy 31:8, NIV)

> *Let the beloved of the Lord rest secure in him, for he shields him [or her] all day long, and the one the Lord loves rests between his shoulders.* (Deuteronomy 33:12, NIV)

I was learning to be grateful for the constant love and strength I found in the encouragement of those who loved me and spoke God's Word to me. The latter always gave me secure rest and a shield from emotional pain. Many times I would lift my hurts, tears, and frustrations to God and begin to praise and lift words of adoration to Him who was so worthy to receive it. In those times, God would sweep in with His peace and warm comfort.

Found Children

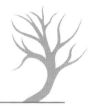

Cassia was our dream child, conceived only in our imagination. For my husband and me, the qualities we valued in a child wouldn't be claimed in our own offspring. God *was* unfolding a wonderful gift in our lives, but I didn't know it at the time.

An amazing thing began to happen when I said yes to a nursery school teaching position in 2007. I loved teaching little people. This very special little school had me hooked during my entrance interview. I took a seat opposite the owner and main teacher in the Montessori and Day Nursery. I was pleasantly amused when, after this husband-and-wife team were seated, their two-year-old son pulled up a chair. His opinion mattered, too!

I must have made an impression, because this began a wonderful relationship with two-year-old Colton, and later his sister Karen whom I met when she was just three hours old. She marked the occasion by pooping on me that first day.

Colton and Karen both made their way through my nursery class and parked themselves permanently in my heart. They attended my summer day camps and enjoyed sleepovers together at our house. Hugs and snuggles became our daily routine for hellos and goodbyes. It was wonderful watching them grow and blossom into the school-age and preteen children they are today.

Eva was two and a half when she tiptoed into my nursery class and simultaneously crawled into my heart. She had a quiet wisdom about her and loved to laugh. She always encouraged me with her smile. Her long blonde hair was fun to pull together into ponytails or pigtails; they often fell apart due to her nervous habit of pulling out strands of hair. Today she is a Kindergarten graduate and is a big sister to another heart-grown child, Emily.

Brothers Carter and Walter stepped into our school boisterous and unafraid. First Carter, then Walter one year later, enjoyed the environment of school and play. Carter was loved immediately by all the girls in Senior Kindergarten while younger brother Walter's quiet personality morphed into comedic energy. Today Carter is the bug man, sharing fascinating facts about all six- or eight-legged creatures. Walter is the weatherman for his family, sharing weather predictions and nature's storms. Both boys share the role of big brother to Little J, the child for whom I enjoyed being nanny for a year.

These three families are found children. They've all come and celebrated a special warm relationship with us. As a couple, we are focused on them. Birthdays, Christmas, playdates, and celebrations are a part of our lives, too! We love them just as we would our own. This is the best tribute we can give in memory of Cassia.

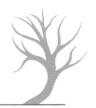

No More Wait in Me

After the intensity of passing our second home study, it felt like everything came to a screeching halt. We waited for a match, a child whose needs we could meet. Once again, we waited and prayed. We felt that we had done everything that was required of us. Though I had found a new hope in a relationship with God, I didn't fully trust Him. After all, I felt that He was withholding something precious from me. I began to believe that certain people got things from God and certain other people didn't qualify. This isn't true, but I began to believe it.

At one point, we found out that our profile had been sent to parents who were choosing adoptive parents for their child. We were thrilled that this could possibly be "the moment." Once again, time passed. We were not chosen. I retreated to that heart-wrenching place of disappointment. To amplify my emotional state, I was dealing with my sister's passing due to breast cancer. It was a low time.

We had sold our home and Dario found work in a nearby city outside the county we had lived in when we started our adoption process with Children's Aid. We were faced with the situation of having to transfer our application to another county and another Children's Aid Society. Dario and I had hope in the process of transferring our file. After all, we had been declared adoption-ready, and all that remained was another home inspection.

Once the new county adoption agency received our file, we eagerly anticipated receiving a request for a meeting. Wanda, our contact, emailed to say that we needed to update our file. This was a normal request, as every two years we had to undergo a police check and vulnerable sectors check. We also had to get complete physicals and letters sent stating the findings. Wanda mentioned beginning a family profile letter and writing pages describing who we were and what we could offer a child. I set to work, as I had always done, attempting to jump through all the hoops. We sent in the paperwork from the local police detachment. I also began to prepare a lovely profile and was happy with the results.

When we moved out of the area, my husband's doctor was nearer, so I switched over as well. I made a phone call one morning to discuss the cost. In the two years prior, the cost for a medical check for a second party was two hundred dollars, so we were prepared somewhat to pay a fee for the doctor's services.

"Yes, good morning," I said when I got on the phone with the doctor's office. "I would like to inquire as to the cost of having a medical done for the Children's Aid Society, for adoption purposes, and to make appointments for both my husband and I."

I took a deep breath, ready to view my calendar for the medical appointment.

The secretary paused long enough to hear my request and then launched into taking our names and securing the appointment. "I believe we could get you and your husband in for subsequent medicals on July 21. One at 1:00 p.m. and the other at 2:00 p.m."

"That sounds great," I said, then added, "And what would be the cost?"

"The cost is three hundred dollars per person, and we accept only cash." The secretary paused again, anticipating my response.

"I don't understand," I said. "Two years ago we paid two hundred dollars. Before we came to see this doctor, I only paid fifty dollars for my second-party medical. How is it possible for the price to jump this much?"

I could feel my pulse race and my face begin to get warm. I had a sinking feeling that this wouldn't go over well with Dario. Calming down, I remembered that Children's Aid had requested this, and in the past they always reimbursed these kinds of fees.

Later that afternoon, I called Wanda, our contact with Children's Aid. I explained the conversation I'd had with our doctor's secretary. Wanda couldn't believe what I told her.

"What? Six hundred dollars in total? We've never had that much money requested for a medical. I'll have to get prior approval before we can reimburse this."

She and I discussed the matter further and decided that I could attempt to call the doctor's office back and ask for a reduction. When I did call back, I explained that it seemed abnormal to ask that much for a medical. My request was met with resistance.

"I don't understand what the Children's Aid contact is talking about," the secretary said. "This is well within the limit of what a doctor can charge for this type of service. We are firm on this fee."

A short time later, our police check paperwork came in and I finished the family profile. Wanda mentioned that the only thing that remained was the medical. We felt we were so close.

Dario and I had been preparing to attend the Adoption Resource Exchange, held a couple of times a year in the Toronto area. We had never gone before because of our adoption status, but now we could attend. I felt like we had qualified. With the paperwork almost completed and our application filled out, we felt it quite natural to cite our town's Children's Aid Society as our adoption worker contact.

Only a day or two after we applied in April 2014, I received an email from Wanda. From what I remember, the email went something like this: "Dear Paula and Dario, I thought it would be important to let you know that when you apply to attend the Adoption Resource Exchange, you cannot yet put down our name as an adoption worker contact as we have not yet accepted you into our Aid Society. You can still attend, but until you are accepted you are without agency representation. Once we receive the medical forms and we have time when our case load is less, we will look at your file."

With no one in the room, I said, "When they have time? When their caseload is less? Does she not get it? We've been waiting seven years!"

I was frantic and Dario was frustrated. I panicked and called our previous adoption worker. She was encouraging and comforting, but said that we were no longer a part of the county we had lived in before, and therefore our file had been closed there. She did offer her name as a temporary contact, but that was all she could offer.

I called the Adoption Resource Exchange director and explained our situation. She listened and offered her comfort as well. She encouraged us to still attend and commented that really someone should go to bat for us. Someone should step up to the plate.

I felt spent. In so many ways, I felt that I just couldn't fight anymore. Yes, I could push and insist that we go, but I felt it would be incredibly cruel to find a little person in the video files and have no opportunity to even put in our request. I was tired of climbing uphill, exhausted in my attempts to make it happen. I had no more wait left in me, and I felt that my world, our lives, meant nothing. No one cared.

We were still waiting. It had been over seven years.

The misunderstanding with our family physician caused us to soul-search, and at that time were facing the painful reality of our preparedness to parent at age fifty. We were looking at the possibility of just letting God take control and release this area of desire and fear of childlessness. From the moment I'd married my husband, I had taken charge of the child-producing process. I had never considered what God's ultimate plan was. He is faithful to always ensure we have strength for the journey and that His love can carry us through every sorrow.

We were at a crossroads. One path was marked "our plan" and the other was marked "His plan." Which one would we take? What would it take to let it go?

After seven years of setbacks, I'd had enough. We decided to close our file for adoption. I cancelled my appointment for my medical and switched doctors. I emailed both Children's Aid Societies and never received an acknowledgement of this closure. No "I'm sorry," no "All the best." Nothing. I was defeated and crushed.

There were so many ifs in my life. If I had gotten married in my twenties, perhaps my ovaries would have responded to the hormone replacement therapy. If I had gotten married earlier, perhaps I could have had luteinizing hormone and follicle-stimulating hormone replacement therapy to balance my body and I could have produced an egg. Perhaps if I was younger, I could have qualified for in vitro fertilization. If we had been affluent and had the money to purchase this process at over ten thousand dollars per try, we might have been parents by now. If only God had healed my body just as He had promised…

At home one afternoon, these thoughts pushed me over the edge. A hot tidal wave of tears and pent-up hopelessness released a fissure of pain. I looked for something to destroy, and the only thing I could do was kick, shred, punch, and rip apart an entire case of toilet paper. I screamed and cried, aiming it all at God. I bawled and shouted, "How unfair You've been to me! Why did You promise and not come through? Why couldn't You have intervened sooner? What was all this for?" I sobbed out years of sorrow in the silence of our country rental home.

My life and faith were in crisis. I had abused God's grace. I had made having a child an idol in my life. I was finished and needed God—and God met me there. Immersed in His mercy (not to mention shredded toilet paper), I was secured by His grace and soothed by His love. I was exactly where God wanted me to be. I had surrendered. I was in His arms.

I learned the lesson that God's way is not only the best way, but the only way. In His mercy, many things have been restored to me. I had a release in my heart, a new peace. My husband and I are making plans again in our lives. Possibilities and choices are blooming all around us. We have chosen to live child-free, and to consider those children who are already in our lives.

I had been looking at what I could do, should do, and would do… if this or that. The truth is that I had felt the pain of regret in this journey of infertility and adoption pursuits. I looked at the past years of my marriage and realized that I hadn't spent one moment just "being." I had been so consumed with trying to make a family that I didn't live life.

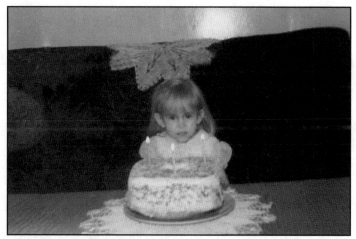

At age three I was barely tall enough to see over my cake!

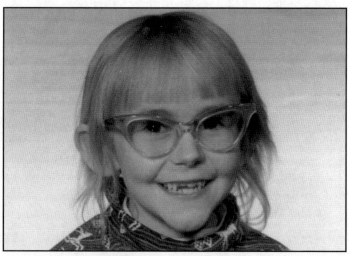

Six years old, just starting school

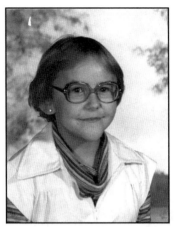

Sweet sixteen - the year I made Jesus my Lord

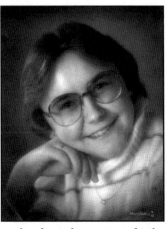

Smiling through sadness, discovering infertility at age 19

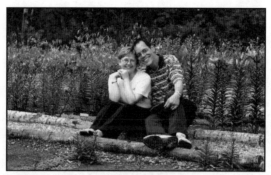

Engaged! I finally found my best friend on earth!

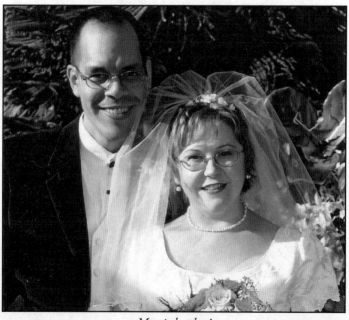

Married at last!

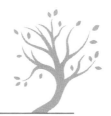

From Mother to Mother

I'm redefining the word "mother." Actually, I'm discovering what the God of the Bible has to say about the definition of "mother" in the way that the authors (read: God) have used the word. I always assumed that the word was defined only as one who's given birth to a son or daughter; with a bit of stretch, maybe it also included legal adoption.

As an inquisitive person, I love to research. The thought occurred to me to hunt out the word "mother" in terms of its Greek or Hebrew origins. I headed straight for the Strong's Concordance. I was so shocked to find that "mother," in the original Hebrew (517), meant "*em*, a primitive word meaning a mother (as in the bond of the family) in a wide sense and used figuratively."[2] This is an Old Testament translation. In the New

[2] James Strong, *The New Strong's Exhaustive Concordance of the Bible* (Nashville, TN: Thomas Nelson, 1995), 10. Hebrew section.

Testament, the Greek word for mother is *meter* (3384), meaning the same thing. Reeling with the possibilities, I searched *Vine's Expository Dictionary of the Bible*. Was it possible that God had already answered my prayer to be a mother by His definition? In Vine's, the word "mother" is defined this way: "of the natural relationship, and figuratively of one who takes the place of a mother."[3]

Jesus referred to this open definition in Mark 3:34–35.

And he looked round about on them which sat about him, and said, Behold my mother and my brethren! For whosoever shall do the will of God, the same is my brother, and my sister, and mother. (KJV)

I am not a Bible scholar and do not claim to be a teacher, but by this definition anyone who nurtures, teaches, and trains a child has already experienced motherhood. As my pastor once told me, although I have never given birth to a child, I have a mother's heart. Knowing that God thinks so, too, gives me much hope.

This Bible verse is still one of my favourites:

He maketh the barren woman to keep house, and to be a joyful mother of children. Praise ye the Lord. (Psalm 113:9, KJV)

---

[3] W.E. Vine, Merrill F. Unger, and William White Jr., *Vine's Complete Expository Dictionary of Old and New Testament Words* (Nashville, TN: Thomas Nelson, 1996), 418.

That word "mother" in this verse is the Greek word *meter*. As I write this, I'm amazed that this definition was here all along. God's plan for me included mothering those who crossed my path, those who in one way or another inherited me in their mother's place at certain times. In God's eyes, He had already answered my prayers. You see, by His definition, in addition to referring to the family relationship, mother is also defined as one who takes the place of a mother. I mother children every day and have wonderful relationships with many.

With this hope, I can breathe, grieve the past, deal with the here and now, and once again trust God to take care of me my whole life through. Any woman who has nurtured a child through providing childcare, hugging a niece or nephew, giving guidance as a coach, or giving love to any child qualifies as a mother. He cares for me and He cares for you. It doesn't change the baby cravings in our hearts; that is simply part of being female. God wants to bring fresh hope to aching hearts and fresh encouragement to those who find it hard to face another day. You and I will make it. He has given us great peace.

I'm also looking at the future. I think there will be a large empty place where I cannot love, comfort, guide, and parent another little person who is wonderfully mine. I also wonder what it would look like, and how the end would be, without anyone being there for us, making decisions for our elder care, or holding our hands as we slip into eternity. I also grieve that there will not be a little Cassia waiting for us in heaven, as those who have had miscarriages can hope for. There is a certain rawness of emotion in knowing that we have to let go of our own plans. Those plans were for a younger version of ourselves with more resources. Yes, I have been sad. I have experienced sadness that caused me to retreat and come up for air just enough to focus on work, our home, and our church. I have held it at bay for now, although at times I weep for what could have been. I'm concentrating on smiling for and with others, because my friendships are important.

Shortly after this new revelation, I visited a church with a friend. No one knew me there. I decided to respond to the call to the front for anyone wanting a touch from the Lord. I have almost never refused an opportunity for prayer and time with the Lord.

I went forward. To my utter shock, the pastor of the church prayed a simple prayer and gave me this word: "The Lord wants you to know that you have been a good mother. He wants you to know that He is so proud of you for being such a good mother. He is pleased that you have been a good mother to many in your life. The Lord wants you to know that you are not a disappointment to Him. You have not disappointed the Lord. He is so proud of you."

This confirming word brought me new comfort, and I felt a final brick slide into place in the tower of strength God was building for me. For once in my life, I felt that God had answered my prayers and I was happy.

Now, each Mother's Day is different. In 2014, I made a clear decision to give honour where it was due. All of God's creation is worthy of celebration, whether these little ones are mine or not. The Lord is teaching me to always return to the place of peace and rest, to keep my empty hands open before the Lord in an open stance. It's a place of surrender and release, working past emotion and casting my cares on Him and giving Him praise in spite of how I feel.

First of all, I will honour my own mother. Although my own mother is far away, across the miles, I'm planning to have a long chat with her and just enjoy her for those moments that I still can. This day is about her, not me!

Secondly, I will celebrate the mothers all around me who show me why I wanted kids in the first place. I go to church and enjoy the people who have become like a second family to me. I will enjoy watching them be blessed as they receive special prayer for what they do day in and day out. I will pray for them, too, and pray for every precious gift that was given to them. On this Mother's Day I will sow (maybe in tears, for the gift that is certain to come to me. It's okay if I have a good cry; God understands the longings of my heart.

Thirdly, I will remember that I'm not damaged goods. I will remember that infertility is what has happened to my body, but it is not who I am. I am the precious daughter of our Heavenly Father." All my peace comes from Him.

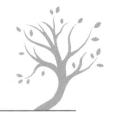

Lost and Found

For us, Cassia and her creation in our hearts and imaginations has become an icon to what infertility has meant to us. She is real in our memories, a representation of what we have lost. She has lived in our imagination and died in our surrender. This book speaks to that loss in a million ways. I am reminded of her almost daily.

Earlier in 2014, I turned our additional bedroom into a music room and office for my reading and writing and other projects. I replaced the bookshelf with a leather chair. I replaced the toy shelf with a medium desk and chair. The dresser now contains my winter clothing instead of the plastic storage bins I had been using. We were able to move my husband's keyboard and music to a side wall. The room is full and its earlier appearance as a child's room is fading from memory.

It was an important process, and in a sense a healing one. As I was clearing out toys and other items, I noticed a plastic pouch. I carefully unzipped the pouch, and to my amazement found a small woollen suit. The leggings and socks where all one knitted piece; they were pink and new looking. The sweater was a perfect match with attached knitted hood. I had found it years ago at a yard sale. It was so tiny and I'd seen that it had hardly been worn. I bought it at a time when my dreams were still real in my heart, years before I was even married.

It seemed so odd now to know that this little sweater had never been worn by Cassia. The odd part was that I felt no pain, no hurt, and no tears—just a little quiet as I fingered the soft knitting. I did, however, feel a bit foolish. I had believed that I could control my own future simply by owning it and expecting it. When I couldn't make our dream come true, I set about manipulating God and others. I'm ashamed at my response to God, expecting a baby out of God's vending machine if I put in enough faith coinage. When all my efforts didn't work, I grieved.

I have learned that all grief has an expiry date, only it is often unknown to others and to oneself. No one can tell you when that is and how long it will take to "get over it." The key is to get up each morning and, regardless of the type of grief, keep reminding yourself to breathe.

Sometimes what is lost needs to stay lost, and what is found needs to stay found—and celebrated. You need to know the difference.

The Other Mother

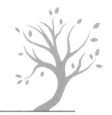

Motherhood has so many faces. Mother's Day is even for those who have given birth but for one reason or another have had to give that baby up for a better future.

I am the "other mother." Each day I put everything I am into nurturing children. I care for a classroom of one- and two-year-olds. All are special relationships. I'm happy that over the years I have had many special relationships with the children in my life as a nursery teacher, Sunday school teacher, and educational assistant. In fact, in June 2014 I celebrated twenty-five years as an early childhood educator. The children I have taught over the years have become "my" children. People used to be shocked when I'd reply that I had eleven children, depending on the number I had in my class each year.

Through one of these special relationships, I received one of the best gifts ever. Ironically, it was a Mother's Day present:

a simple poem written by a grateful mom on a colourful card cut in the shape of her five-year-old son's hand. Accompanying this card was a clay handprint of her one-year-old daughter. The card read, "You're our 'Other Mother', you've been there from the start. We didn't grow in your tummy, we grew right in your heart." I have kept that simple, honest, heartfelt gesture of love for many years now and I never get tired of rereading it. These heart-grown children will always stay, no matter how old they get. With each new year comes new additions of special children, causing my heart to expand.

I suppose that if I were to describe motherhood, I'd describe the nurturing love that "other mothers" have though they may or may not have ever given birth. "Other mothers" love other children and take the time to build special relationships with love and playfulness, affection and interest. They find ways to support and encourage children's growth with each interaction.

Who are these "other mothers"? They are your friends who offer weeknights to watch your children while you enjoy a well-deserved date night. They are your children's nursery, Kindergarten, and Sunday school teachers who dry tears and soothe owies while you're at work or in church. They include the elderly lady who never married, who lives next door and always puts extra treats in your children's bag at Halloween. These are women who never had children, but love yours. These "other mothers" are all around you. How will you show them your love and appreciation next Mother's Day?

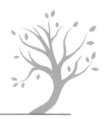

Assumptions

In many ways, we all make assumptions as we carry on throughout the day. We assume things about the people around us. We assume that the beat-up truck in front of us must be owned by a poor person. Or we think to ourselves that the clerk at the checkout is rude and doesn't like her job because she snapped at the customer in front. The child in the grocery store is throwing a wild tantrum in aisle three and the mother does nothing. She must be a terrible mother.

We've all been there, whether we voice these assumptions or not.

Some assumptions can sting a little, as I have recently discovered. It was a sunny day and finally I was able to take the little toddler I was caring for that day out for a morning stroll and window shopping. We really were having a lovely time in the clothing department, checking out clearance items and making animal noises to match the many cute animal t-shirts.

I didn't notice her at first, being so entranced by a kitty t-shirt priced at only $7.99. This woman was mesmerized by the sweet boy I held in hand. She eyed me, then gazed at the blue-eyed charmer, then glanced back at me.

"Well hello," she said.

I eagerly said hello. This seemed to give her permission to press me further in order to confirm her assumption. Her gaze caught the eye of the busy boy at my feet.

"Are you out for some shopping time with Grandma?" she asked.

In my visits to an Early Years Centre with this little boy I nanny, I enjoy the romp and play of all the other "littles" as they embark on their first discoveries of play group. I get to rub shoulders with moms and their infants and toddlers. It's a wonderful atmosphere. It's also a place where many assume I am the mommy, or at least grandma, to this adorable toddler. It sometimes makes me feel the secret pleasure of being part of the "mommy group." I now realize how left out I'd felt for thirty years. I now belonged, even in omission of the truth. Someone once said, "It is better to remain silent and be thought a fool than to open your mouth and remove all doubt."

As an early childhood educator, there is much I can contribute to a conversation regarding young children, and I enjoy doing so.

I didn't see it coming this time.

Without warning, one day while amongst the mommy group, I was asked a question that only mothers ask other mothers: "How long were you in labour?"

The room went from warm loving candour to the hot rushing heat of embarrassment.

"Actually I'm the nanny," I said. "Little J is my work. We were never able to have children."

The conversation stilled to a too-long pause and calmly shifted to the unimportant facts and details of life reserved for those outside the club. "What strange weather we're having…" I was no longer part of *them*.

To explain the other side of assumptions, perhaps that beat-up truck in the lane in front of you was purchased by an affluent mechanic. Perhaps he was determined to fix it for his next-door neighbour, a single mother who walks across town to get to her hotel-cleaning job after the kids get picked up by the school bus. Perhaps it was to be a surprise gift after it was cleaned and repaired.

Perhaps that clerk at the checkout who snapped at a customer just discovered this morning that her husband was having an affair. Perhaps she just couldn't take one more moment of hiding her broken heart.

That child throwing a tantrum? Perhaps the mom's not a bad mother but has just buried her husband of seven years due to a car accident and she's still numb. It's only been a month.

Those who love children are not all mommies. A simple solution for inquiring minds is to merely ask, "How are you connected to this beautiful child?" It's the type of question anyone can answer without any awkward moments or incorrect supposition. Or so I assume…

Beware of the Little Clouds

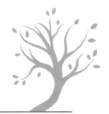

"Yes, Little J, we're going for a car ride. C'mon, we're a little late."

Our Tuesday morning routine always includes a trip to the Early Years Centre. As we made our way to my vehicle one day, the sun matched my optimistic outlook. The slight breeze and clear sky projected a perfect morning. Only one small cloud threatened to take it all away.

Arriving just in time for circle time, Little J and I found our places on the play rug. The songs and story were always fun, and we joined in with jubilant singing. Little J jumped up at its conclusion and headed for the snack room. He scampered ahead of me to find his place at the table and settled in with apples, cheese cubes, and frosted cereal. Once the small group of children were seated and snacks had been distributed, I joined the moms.

I always loved the rich conversation I could be part of with the moms there. These were discussions of temper tantrums, how to cut a two-year-old's hair, and how to get an older sibling's bubble gum out of the family pet's fur. These were discussions of life that could include all participants. Sandra, mom of eighteen-month-old Corinna, nursed her coffee. Debbie, mother of three with two-and-a-half-year-old Jason, had the habit of chewing nervously on her inner cheek. Today she was tuning in to what Sandra had to say. Today's discussion was about Sandra's obstetrician.

"I've been happy with Dr. Ruby," Sandra said. "She was the one who helped me birth Corinna here. With my first, I had the other doctor."

Debbie nodded in agreement and quickly saved her son's cereal from dumping to the floor before speaking. "Didn't she take over from Dr. Smythe? She was my first OB. She was really nice."

Sandra shook her head. "I didn't think she had a lot of personality. I found her hard to relate to."

"Yeah," Debbie replied. "She seemed kind of disinterested until it was time to give birth. Then she was very nurturing and kind. She came alive then."

I had been listening to this conversation with feigned interest and without comment. The next statements got my attention.

Sandra looked at me for a split second, then at Debbie. "Well, I have to go in to see Dr. Ruby. She has to put in my IUD." An IUD is an intrauterine device, used for contraception.

Debbie had a smile on her face. "She put mine in recently. I didn't feel badly at all."

I felt badly at that moment. Part of me wanted to cry out, "That is so unfair. There are so many women who would give their left arm to be given the chance to conceive at will, and you just dismiss it like a menu option." I didn't say a single word, as it's not my place to comment on the decisions of others. Thankfully, Little J was finished and I ushered him out of the snack area toward the play room. The room was darkened by the clouds ushering in a thunderstorm only moments away.

I knew that this method of contraception was on the rise in Canada. In the 1970s, it received a bad rap for causing inflammatory disease due to a flaw in its design. Seemingly, that flaw had been resolved as it was now deemed fit to use. The effectiveness is good: apparently only one out of a hundred women will get pregnant.

This sounds like the odds of those experiencing infertility. To illustrate how unfair health insurance can be, the Merena, a hormone-releasing version of contraception that ensures pregnancy cannot occur, is covered by most private health insurance plans in Canada. The irony is that an IVF treatment isn't covered by private health insurance plans in Canada. It's not considered a medically necessary treatment.

Why do these conversations bring out the right and wrong in me? My inner-wisher would like to tell the world that not everyone can handle a conversation like this, and I can only imagine how a woman undergoing IVF treatment would be wounded to overhear this natter. Yet I know they were speaking in their innocence and out of their own worldview. I would like the world to know that sometimes it would be nice for a little sensitivity when conversing about such intimacies in public. You never know whom you might hurt.

Thankfully, I wasn't wounded by this discussion. Little J and I decided that lunch was a far more interesting affair and we made our way to Little J's home. By the time we parked in the driveway, my sunshine day was gone and the clouds had released their burden.

There is a defining moment, I think, when every person comes to a crossroads in their life. It doesn't matter what the issue is. It could be a relationship, change of employment, or terminating attempts to conceive or adopt. Normally there is a catalyst for a decisive moment to occur—the straw that broke the camel's back, so to speak.

These moments come to all of us at some point, or even several times in one's life. One moment you're travelling along in a clearly defined direction, then in the next moment the road separates into unknown paths requesting—no, demanding—a decision. It's a time when what you thought so clearly defined you becomes the very thing that condemns you. The threat of living without the object of your desire becomes very, very real.

Living Child-Friendly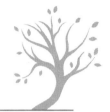

Freedom and resolution to infertility come in a number of ways. The obvious way is that a child becomes your very own through conception, a wonderful gift and one that should be sought with every effort. Adoption is another way to start a family. It is not for everyone, but for those it fits, it is a wonderful blessing. I didn't know there was a third option. I didn't understand that living child-free, for some, could be a fulfilling journey.

Since my husband and I made the decision to discontinue our adoption process, I have been intrigued by the various terminologies out there to describe couples without children.

Some couples are still grieving the loss that infertility brings; having exhausted their efforts, they have decided that they are "childless." This term has always saddened me because it implies permanent loss. I don't believe it has to be that way.

Other couples have come to a place of giving up on all the pain of infertility and its medical processes and have decided that they are "child-free." Although this implies a certain freedom, I have always felt a bit uncomfortable with this label as it implies that children are no longer a part of life, and almost a group to be disliked.

I have found a better word to describe the journey that I'm on, the one I have penned my story about in this book: "child-friendly."

You see, right from when I was a small child I have wanted to be a mommy. I played that way and talked that way until my diagnosis. Discovering your infertility when you're single is a double whammy! You cannot discover or do anything about it. One thing, however, became clear: I had a prolific sibling group. This meant that beloved nieces and nephews were everywhere, and I loved them.

Children became part of my daily existence, so much so that I chose early childhood education as a career. I always thought I'd have my own one day. To me, motherhood is the greatest employment and greatest ministry. I will always have great respect for those who accept this call.

Children will always be important to me. The concept of living child-free implies that I will have no children in my life. As this was not my desire, I prefer to live child-friendly. Semantics? Maybe, but for me it fits.

My husband and I warmly accept children into our home and we celebrate graduation from Kindergarten, birthdays, and Christmas with them. Sharing gifts, activities, and cake with them are joys to us as well. We love to see their faces light up when we can share a part of their lives.

There's no big punchline or wonderful end to this choice. It's a special part of our lives. I am sure that one day I will find a place where these relationships can bloom and blossom into lifetime joys, but I'm not responsible for that. I will walk and bless the next child in front of me, whomever it may be: a neighbour's boy, a great niece, a child at church, or a little girl who stares at me in Wal-Mart, I am living content. I am the "other mother" to many. For this I am grateful.

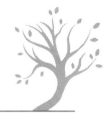

Who Am I to Become?

Living "child-friendly" has given me much to think about. In one way or another, I find myself grateful for the extra time, and the freedom to choose. I find that my mind is no longer overcome by fears and what-ifs and the whens and hows. I'm in the throes of living a quiet, contented life. Living in peace from the stresses of pre-adoption and wondering why my body won't obey the simple command to multiply and replenish the earth is something I only hoped for in the past.

I am working to put all that behind me. The pain of being called a grandma when I held the hand of my two-year-old charge, or waiting and waiting for yet another delay in the adoption process to be resolved, are almost forgotten. I almost wonder if I will ever completely forget.

As I find new peace in this surrender, I find my God. He is my greatest Friend. Fear of failure and loss of control resurface from time to time. I have to learn to overcome fear through my a love walk with God the Father. I cannot fail, because my loss of control puts God in control. This is far better.

In this process, another question rises to the surface of my soul: who am I now? In the past, I was infertile. Since I'm not attempting to conceive, does this condition stick? I was also pre-adoptive. Since I'm not attempting to adopt, who am I?

I can live, and I can love, but I am not defined. I can be the woman God is creating me to be, and the latter half of my life is full of potential.

Every day I look deeply into the eyes of the children I work with and make a special effort to really see and connect with them. Once a six-year-old said to my employer, "I love Paula because she loves me." She was asked, "Why do you think Paula loves you?" The little girl replied, "Because she treats us like we are her own kids!" There is no greater compliment.

A new identity? Child-friendly? This describes my outlook and my way of reaching out. Who am I? I am His. The great God-Jehovah holds my hand.

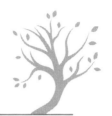

Such a Simple Question

The colourfully illustrated book caught my attention as the toddler I care for manipulated its pages. The pictures were beautifully drawn and displayed a woman in various stages of pregnancy and childbirth. In the midst of coming to terms with how I view motherhood, according to the biblical definition, this issue was so much a part of me that I found reminders everywhere. I had been thinking about infertility and how I had been enduring a much-too-long wait to have a child through adoption.

The book's title was *Where Do Babies Come From?* It seems like a simple question. All that seems to be needed to answer the question is a wish, a desire, and the physical union of one unsuspecting egg to one very determined little sperm swimmer. However, for those experiencing infertility, the answer isn't quite that simple.

Ladies who cannot conceive the normal way have chosen to begin families with the many possibilities out there that *may* succeed, from the various methods of natural conception (the basal temperature method, the cervical mucus method, and the calendar method all help to detect when you're most fertile) to science-aided methods (intrauterine insemination, in vitro fertilization, sperm-donor shopping, and surrogate motherhood) and all the way to the adoption of waiting children. Still, one would think this would be easy. For a lot of us, it's not.

The promises of God encourage the barren to sing (Isaiah 54) and for women to be the happy mother of children (Psalm 113:9). He also promises to heal broken bodies (Hebrews 11:11). Looking at faith this way encourages one to believe in the supernatural rather than the normal means of conception. Still, there is a struggle.

So where do babies come from? Is it human effort? Certainly human cooperation is involved. Is it a blessing from God? A healing to be grasped? Is the fruit of the womb His reward (Psalm 127: 3) Are these based on faith in God or human effort or both?

There is always a plan. God always has a plan to use His power. We can choose medical methods, if that works for us and they are enhanced by His power to heal. He alone knows the unfolding of that plan in our lives. Our response is to trust. This is the authentic enquiry. Can I trust Him? Could I trust Him enough to move on into a child-friendly lifestyle, that includes removing my preparations for Cassia? This was the true test, and it was not a simple question for me. I had to come face to face with this decision.

This Is It!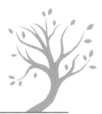

There came a time when I needed to set about cleaning and reorganizing my second bedroom. I wasn't sure if putting it off meant I had actually made the decision or just stopped the craziness of waiting for a child. It had been a long process to get where I am today.

I had been in the process of reorganizing the bedroom, but I finally moved some things out to signify that the decision was final. We were moving forward and had decided to stop trying to find a child for our family. We had decided that we already were a family, my husband and I.

I began with the chest of drawers that held blankets and extra bedding for the single bed in the corner. Some I gave away and some I kept in the cedar chest for company. I removed the rocking chair into another part of the house for the sheer joy of reading. I boxed and stored some toys, which I'll decide to give to whomever I choose, or I may use them in my classrooms.

I adjusted the location of a new penholder several times on my writing desk. No corner or area seemed fitting. All was going well.

Then I looked heavenward to the top of a bookshelf—and there he was: a small fuzzy chocolate-brown bear with big brown eyes and a sad pout. His expression seemed to be mourning the change in me and the function of the room. "What are you doing?" he seemed to ask.

I was shocked how loud his imaginary voice sounded to my ears and the immediate sense of guilt his voice implied.

"I… um… I'm just cleaning a little and moving a few things into storage," I stammered.

"Well, I'm sure glad to see that cabbage patch doll get boxed. She was so annoying. Where did the other things go and what happened to the rocking chair?"

"Well, Mr. Bear, I'm reorganizing things to make this room more purposeful. You see, it's time to move on. My husband and I are becoming child-friendly."

The stunned silence that followed gave me the opportunity to contemplate whether or not this curious little bear needed a place to rest for the time being in the special plastic box I kept for stuffies. I wondered how this fuzzy friend would handle it. Seeing my chance, I snatched the bear, but he somehow missed my grasp and tumbled to the floor.

"Hey, that hurt! Pick me up! Put me back! Put me back!" the bear screamed in my head.

"Okay, little bear, simmer down. You know, you've stood by me and our children's bedroom things for seven years now. You've grown a little dusty and a little cranky. It's time to put aside this constant struggle of finding a child. We cannot put our lives on hold inevitably. It's time to let go. This room will be a music room and office now."

"A… a… are you letting go of m… m… me?" he asked. His imploring eyes impacted my heart.

I thought for a moment. I'd held him in my hands far too long. I couldn't just let him go, could I? He stood for my hopes and dreams. He had been with me a long time and I couldn't just toss him in a plastic box for storage. Yet I had a rule that all my things had to serve a purpose. It suddenly seemed cruel. Two little bears appeared on each of my shoulders, whispering opposing views. One carried a tiny pitchfork while the other had angel wings. I brushed them off and returned to gaze at the bear's frozen stare.

"You and I have been together a long time, haven't we, buddy?" At this, his tiny face softened. I squeezed him close.

Enough cleaning for now, I thought as I placed the bear down.

Walking out of the room, I smiled. This little brown bear will always remind me of the struggle and pain and cost of infertility. Looking at him, I realized that I cannot file it all away and put it out of my mind. This would be a process… a slow letting go of what was, a grieving of what could have been.

For now, my little brown bear sits smugly on my desk, almost clutching the penholder there. He, too, has a purpose. He fits perfectly.

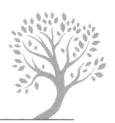

Looking Back

Infertility doesn't define who I am. It is a journey I have travelled through a large portion of my life, but it is not me.

The bizarre thing is that living with infertility has its own progression. It's not just about the discovery, diagnosis, and medical process. It's not about the requirements of adoption, paperwork, interviews, and waiting. The journey of infertility has brought me to turn full-face on myself.

When infertility came into my world at nineteen, I still had a lot of wait left in me. I waited twenty-one years to be married, so the frustration of my body not working properly seemed difficult, but I had time. Yet as I aged, I always felt as though I was running out of time. Just before I was married, I looked at medical options and hoped for a healing. When I actually married, I thought surely I would get pregnant on my honeymoon. I actually had maternity clothing and baby clothes. Furnishings and children's toys came later in my wait.

You see, in the past I have struggled with the need to be in control. I have needed to know everything in advance. I needed to understand how things work and why (or why not). I needed to know the implication of every decision and then decide accordingly. I needed to control things so I could change the deep unhappiness inside me. Yet time and time again, I found myself in surrender.

One day in May, I planned to have a great morning at church. During the worship, I felt the familiar fear and panic rise up. I felt failure, longing, and hopelessness as I looked around at the families with children. In that moment, I couldn't fight back the tears, so I ran for cover into the bathroom, my crying place.

That same morning at prayer, I sat cross-legged in front of the pulpit and poured out my heart. I prayed to God, saying that I wanted to live in His will, and I opened my hands to let my desire drop to the floor. I wept for what I couldn't produce for my husband and sobbed for wanting things my way. The Lord comforted and cleansed me right there. There, very tentatively, I asked the Lord to remove the pain of desire for children and allow Him to answer that prayer in the way He chose.

My longing for a child was insatiable. In all my praying and waiting and testing, I didn't find any peace. I had time, I thought. After all, I was only forty-one, forty-two, forty-three… The frustration mounted as I fought with issues of being unable to control my body, regardless of how much I commanded it to change. I certainly knew I wasn't in control. One could almost hear the clock ticking softly.

My personal clock suddenly stopped ticking the day I discovered I didn't qualify for IVF treatments. I had to be ushered into a side room in order to gain emotional control. I had to stay in control. When that avenue closed, I threw myself into painful prayer. If I prayed exactly right and prayed the right scriptures repeatedly, God would owe me a baby. I would pace and pray, speaking aloud to God exactly what I expected Him to do.

After a full year of this futility, I called the adoption agency and we began an eight-year process. I had renewed hope that surely this was the reason we couldn't have children; we were called to adopt! The enthusiasm didn't last long. After only a year of paperwork and meetings, we were put on hold. In a few years we would be called to begin the process of classes and home study, but there was time for that. We waited. We jumped through more hoops and waited again.

When spring came, a new announcement from the adoption agency brought me to a place of renewed strength and determination that this time I could take control by surrender. We could decide when enough was enough.

Keyboard and page cannot possibly record all that my husband and I have invested through the years of this emotional, physical, and pain-filled attempt to conceive or adopt a child. I was exhausted and ready to let the dream go.

I owe a lot of heartfelt thanks to my pastors, Robert and Brenda Powell, for their countless moments of love, prayer, and counsel. I will forever be grateful. I was ready to surrender not just the dream, but my need to control. I was ready to let God take over.

He did! In letting go, I have found a new sense of peace. It has been an incredible relief to be free of the torment. No, I haven't found a baby on my doorstep or snatched a toddler at the mall. I don't intend to. I'm learning to live free—child-friendly free. Knowing that I'm already a mother in the lives of many little ones, I can rest and walk in God's design for me. I am a mother in place of another.

From the time of diagnosis to the day of surrender, I have been trading time and effort in a bargain with God. He patiently waited and gave me the time to discover that He has always been in control. This, for me, was a moment of release. I would know that God had healed me when I could rejoice at a Mother's Day church service without feeling pain and anguish.

This journey may not be over. I don't know what tomorrow will bring or what the future will hold. This is a journey I've travelled, but it's not who I am.

Empty Hands to Open Arms

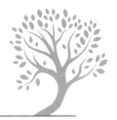

Infertility has given us all empty hands that were meant to be filled with a little boy or girl. It is a place of vulnerability. A person can feel so weak when they have nothing to give, feeling emptiness that those who have searched for answers and have not found them.

The term "open arms" has a twofold meaning to me. It speaks of our openness to support, lift, and encourage one another in this journey to resolution, whatever that may be. It may be that your open arms will embrace a child, and for others it may be the open arms to embrace the childless. "Open arms" also speaks of our openness to God, His plan, and the unfolding of His will, whatever that may be. We can feel the hope, expectancy, and strength to move forward in the resolution God brings us.

Some may wonder if I still believe in healing. Yes, I do, without reservation. I believe that Jesus gave us the greatest example of the Father's will regarding healing. For me, I believe I couldn't receive that gift because of continual bouts of emotional upheaval. I couldn't trust. Time wasn't in my favour and I was consumed with wanting to control God. I operated in unbelief and blame when my works program didn't move God.

I have in my life received other healing easily. Having lost some hearing in my right ear, one day after receiving prayer it popped and I was able to hear clearly. This was documented at a hearing test a month later; I could hear perfectly. During prayer another time, God touched my left jaw and miraculously replaced some cartilage in my socket, cushioning my temporomandibular joint. God was able to touch me without me being in the way. I let go, and when I did, Jesus moved in my life. Having said that, there are some things we may never know on this side of heaven. God is sovereign and He knows what hinders us.

I See You Everywhere: An Imagined Scenario

Her eyes lifted, momentarily from the *Parenthood* magazine she encased her emotions behind. In the quiet waiting room of the infertility clinic, we barely noticed one another. All I heard was the soft buzz of activity at the nursing station and the calls answered by a rushed receptionist attempting to book yet another patient. Hasty physicians walked briskly from room to room, giving pause to a quickly opened file; they would sigh and walk into each room to deliver verdicts.

The woman was young, possibly twenty-five years on this earth. The ring on her finger showed that she would have to face the verdict alone. Would the news of her fate elicit courage or tears? All was kept secret behind a pretty face by Maybelline, and soft auburn hair combed down. She clutched a silver and black Coach purse as tightly as she clung to her tense, nervous composure. Her eyes reflected the only question she was poised to ask: "Why?"

Our small company of two grew to four as a mother and her cradled newborn entered the room. The mother was completely oblivious to the two women who regarded her bundle. She peeled back a bright pink cotton blanket to reveal another tiny sleeper wrapping her resting child. It was this mom's moment to share her prize with the medical team. The child's face was relaxed in perfect peace. The baby's long lashes, tiny nose, and perfect pink lips reflected the perfect creation she was. The mother held this darling close to her heart.

I glanced at the childless woman and thought I heard the small, cool intake of breath. I saw in her eyes the longing, mixed with a painful mist clouding her blue eyes, which turned a watery shade of grey. I knew that look. I knew the constricting of the heart as pain seared emotions inadequately shared with someone, anyone who understood. In these moments, small bits of joy are smothered in the reality of unanswered dreams and unanswered questions.

Instinctively, I wanted to reach over, grab her hand, place an arm around her burdened shoulder, and whisper that I understood. I yearned to reach to the depth of her hurting heart and soothe the ache there, to tell her it really would be okay, that there was a resolution to be found and comfort to come. However, I hadn't been given the privilege to enter her world. Hurts that deep can only be shared with deep trust in one who listens without giving insensitive advice.

Only a moment later, the woman's name was called and she rose to accept the news. I smiled as our eyes met, and then she was gone.

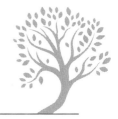

If You've Ever Wondered

I f you've ever wondered about your life and how God could possibly care, you are not alone. For the one who knows this pain, who understands this journey of infertility, from the deep places in me, I grieve for you. At times, when I know your particular struggle, I see the pain that's so familiar. God sees it, too, and Jesus longs to take your hand, put His arms around your hurting heart, and release the burden that is uniquely yours. He longs for you to know that it really will be okay and that He has a resolution for you, when you're ready for it to come into your life. "Hold on to hope," He says. He won't give you insensitive advice. He longs to bring comfort if only you will give Him the privilege to enter your world. Many here on this planet will understand.

So often we struggle with various challenges, and we do so alone. Yet you are not alone. Besides the fact that many people all around you care about what you're going through, you have a God in heaven who cares very much what happens to you. He has chosen to wait as a perfect Gentleman for you to want His help. He won't take over where He has not been invited. He is delighted by you and loves you so deeply. God thinks you are pretty cool, and guess what? He doesn't think you need to earn His love. There's no working for His kindness. You are His favourite. You are the one He misses the most.

He sent Jesus His Son so that all the bad things that have ever happened to you, whether others-inflicted or self-inflicted, would be wiped away. No record of it. Clean slate. He just wants to know if you want it or not.

> *For God so loved the world that he gave his one and only Son, that whoever believes in him shall not perish but have eternal life.* (John 3:16, NIV)

His invitation is simple: "Come." It's easy. Just a little decision. If you call on Him, asking for help, He is there. He's been waiting, longing, and loving you from a distance. Actually, He's only at arm's length, because we are the ones who push Him away. Do you think you have to be perfect to come to Him? You don't. You already are perfect in His eyes. He sees you at your best, even if you don't look that way right now. Just come to Him. The Bible, His book, says *"that if you confess with your mouth the Lord Jesus and believe in your heart that God has raised Him from the dead, you will be saved"* (Romans 10:9–10, NKJV).

"Help, God. I need You!" This is the best prayer ever spoken. You and He can talk about anything. He is listening, He is here, and He is near.

Pray, "Oh God, I am interested in having that clean slate. I know that I've messed up in my life and done wrong. I'm asking for Your help today. I'm asking for You to be my Lord, the Master of my life. I cannot do this alone. From here on in, I want to do things Your way. Help me to know what that is. I believe today that You sent your Son Jesus to pay the price of death that was meant for me. Jesus took away all that I deserved. When I come to You, I can be saved. That means You and I will never be apart from one another ever again. In Jesus' name, amen."

And with that He responds, "My precious child, your faith is equally precious and you are brought closer to Me by your use of it. Keep that faith growing, learning, and trusting. Find your way through applied faith in what I say in My Word, as if it were true, because it *is* true and it has the power of My Father, your Father, to bring about the answers you are looking for. Tell Me about your fears and sorrows. Just as I have freely given to you, receive freely and freely give."

He loves you! Yes, He does.